CW01653376

RoadPeace Poetry

by

Mike Bartram

Grosvenor House
Publishing Limited

This book is published by
Grosvenor House Publishing Ltd
Link House
140 The Broadway, Tolworth, Surrey, KT6 7HT.
www.grosvenorhousepublishing.co.uk

This book is a work of fiction. Any resemblance to people or events, past or present, is purely coincidental.

A CIP record for this book
is available from the British Library

ISBN 978-1-78623-241-0

Dedicated to Bobby Colleran

Foreword

We are honoured and proud that Mike has written such a powerful poetry book dedicated to our beautiful son Bobby. The poems will make people realise the heartbreak & devastation that road accidents cause to victims & their families. I am positive that the poems will make drivers stop, think and realise how much their actions on the road matter.

'Together we can make a difference'

Joanne Colleran

May 2018

Introduction

The death of a loved one in a road crash is a devastating and life changing experience. When Bobby Colleran died in a road crash, his mother vowed to do all she could to prevent the same thing happening to others and she has campaigned tirelessly to help achieve this, through her "Slow Down For Bobby" campaign. Bobby and his mother have inspired Mike to write poetry to raise awareness of the need for everyone who uses our roads to use them responsibly, whether as a driver or a pedestrian. I hope that these poems will make everyone aware of their responsibility on the roads.

Joanne and her family have been supported by RoadPeace, a charity which was founded in 1992 by Brigitte Chaudhry after her son was killed in a road crash. It was set up to provide victims with information, support and practical help with legal proceedings – help that she had not been able to find. RoadPeace offers support through a helpline, befrienders, a resilience building programme and local groups. It also helps with advocacy and casework and it organises remembrance services as it is so important to remember family and friends who have died in a road crash. To find out more about the work of RoadPeace see www.roadpeace.org or telephone the office on 0207733 1603 or the Helpline on 0845 4500 355.

Sincere thanks to Mike for writing this book and to Joanne for all she has achieved.

Pauline Fielding

RoadPeace North West Local Group Coordinator

Contents

RoadPeace

A devastating loss, a life changing day.
Lost in a world of confusion and dismay.
Where was the help, support and care?
In an empty world alone, nobody there.

An 'acceptable death' on road or street.
The kind of response most likely to meet.
A one sided legal system in court to face.
'3rd class victim' attitude was a disgrace.

Dismissed and irrelevant, ignorant of fact.
Parts of the establishment one cosy pact.
Road crime victims reduced to 'fair game'
No understanding to help through the pain.

Things had to change, needed to be done.
And so they were by a road victims Mum.
And so that's how 'RoadPeace' came to be.
All the respect in the world she has from me.

The Snowman

If we get heavy snow and not just rain.
Build a little snowman in Bobby's name.
Don't forget to give it a cheeky like grin!
That'll remind people it was built for him.

Build the greatest snowman in the land!
Get all your best mates to lend a hand.
A snowman who'll be Bobby's namesake.
Deserves to be special, every last flake.

Around his neck wrap an Everton scarf.
Tie it with love on every scousers behalf.
Give him 2 twig arms and a carrot nose.
Give him a warm hug if a cold wind blows.

With a cosy blue hat he will look the part.
Stand back and admire your work of art!
Before you leave him and say 'goodnight'
Give him a kiss on his cheeks pure white.

But if you rise one morning from your bed.
And find that you have a little tear to shed.
As you might discover the sun has shone.
And your Bobby snowman has all but gone.

But remember unlike snow that melts away.
Bobby's loving memory will be here to stay.
As such memories will *never* melt or dim.
The world never forgets a little boy like him.

So please don't cry, not at Christmas time.
Bobby's in Heaven, a light forever to shine.
Because Angels glow he twinkles like a star.
The brightest light in the Festive sky by far.

Crash *Not* Accident

The word 'accident' is so often misused.
It's lazy, its wrong its language abused.
A false impression created with this word.
A denial of the truth, so often not heard.

'Preventable collision' no 'accident' to me.
Accidents do happen, still so sad to see.
But a reckless motorist who causes harm.
Such as driving along with mobile in palm.

Or arrogant drivers, speed limits to break.
Nobody else matters when risks they take.
You can't tell me with behaviour so rash.
The 'accidents' they cause, are *not* a 'crash'

Let It Wait

A crafty look down to their lap.
A message to read, one to tap.
Why does this widely still go on?
Where's the sense, I see none?
I've seen it today, time after time.
Punishment should fit the crime.
A lengthy ban for those caught.
The right lesson has to be taught.
Selfish drivers put lives at stake.
Just for a call to receive or make.
Let it flash, let it bleep, let it wait.
Phone when safe, don't tempt fate.

Living Streets Group

In London's Hackney, a radical twist!
I'd love to see far more of these exist.
A permit granted for a car parking bay.
But it's not getting used in that way!

It's now a 'people parking bay' instead.
Brenda's great idea it has to be said!
For benches or bikes a kerbside space.
A rest spot for walkers, an ideal place.

Most passers-by admire this idea too.
Objections raised, a short sighted few.
Why should the car always dominate?
Living Streets Group want that debate.

As Brenda's idea wasn't council backed.
Understanding for years they have lacked.
But this project deserves the green light.
As people before cars to me seems right.

Broken Heart

Can I swap my heart it's broken beyond repair?
I'm asking God for this, in the form of a prayer.
He must hear a similar prayer every single day.
Sorry if I appear selfish, it's not my usual way.
What I'm asking you for is an impossible task.
But can you *mend* my heart that is all I ask?
Other people who suffer, I feel for their need.
As in this sad world, broken hearts can breed.
But if you get a minute can you look at my case?
As sometimes I wake up to a day I cannot face.

5

I wake up today and ask myself why.
5 people on our roads today will die.
That's the national average in the UK.
And countless more injured each day.
I wonder who those 5 peoples will be.
Could be someone close to you or me.
Unlikely, improbable and thankfully so.
Those figures make the odds very low.
Tragedy close to home may seem rare.
But the fact remains 5 deaths *will* occur.

One Inconsiderate Act

As I read an old account I had a tear in my eye.
An unnecessary death of a child the reason why.
Any death of a child is devastating in every way.
Children are precious and light up our every day.

If such losses are avoidable, greater is the pain.
A needless loss of young life, only Heaven to gain.
I read this young girl died, nearly 50 years ago.
She ran along the pavement, skipping to and fro.

A car blocked her path, left in a dangerous place.
She stepped aside to avoid it, into traffic to face.
A young life lost, because of one inconsiderate act.
If *you* park in such a way, please consider that fact.

Bobby's Light

Every October look up to the sky.
With telescope or just naked eye.
A meteor shower you might see.
A spectacular display it could be.
If the wind blows all clouds away.
And cloudless the night can stay
Then it will be an awesome sight.
A dazzling show through the night
But don't be fooled, easily misled.
If you see lights, blue, green or red.
They may be radiant, that's no lie.
As they aluminate the Autumn sky.
Remember as to the sky you stare.
To Bobby's light they don't compare!

Myth

I think it's a myth, this road we 'share'
Just look around it seems so unfair.
Vehicles dominate, increasingly so.
Pedestrians at times, no place to go.

Make side streets safer for kids to play.
Drivers seem to have all their own way.
Improve public transport, bus and train.
As we 'share' these roads only in name.

Promote shared cars on the school run.
Cycling's another option, if safe it's fun.
Free up the highways from polluted air.
Then we *might* say, the roads we share.

The 'Perfect Driver'

Driving mistakes, there are a common five.
Because nobody is perfect when they drive.
Some of those errors may come as a surprise.
And all mistakes can spell danger in my eyes.

Never use your mobile while the engine is on.
Try and plan your journey time, to and from.
Ignore any in car distractions, let them all wait.
Facts show more drivers crash if running late.

Check your mirrors and keep far enough wide.
There could be cyclists riding on your inside.
Driving on Roundabouts learn the correct drill.
Make your intentions clear is an essential skill.

Keep hydrated, or concentration levels will fall.
Drinking plenty of water keeps you on the ball.
We are all prone to such mistakes on this list.
Because to me the 'perfect driver' doesn't exist.

Road Side Memorials

How far must you travel, not far it seems?
Before you see the site of broken dreams.
Those road side memorials, tragic to see.
Each one, one too many, you must agree.
Another road crash victim, a tragedy born.
Many a crash site, I see flowers to adorn.
Children's toys and teddies, it's hard to take.
One preventable death, so much heartache.
I see trees or lampposts with mementoes tied.
A tearful remembrance for those who died.
Football team colours in form of scarf or crest.
Left in memory for those who peacefully rest.
Think for a moment if you pass such a scene.
Respect and remember just what they all mean.

Deterrent

I'm pleased at the outcome of this high profile case.
A heavy fine it was decided was insufficient to face.
So the driver now faces community service instead.
More Judges should follow this lead; it has to be said.
It's an issue that's been raised many times before.
We should all be treated alike in the eyes of the law.
A deterrent is needed, not just a fine easy to afford.
A deterrent this may prove, so it's a decision I applaud.
Nobody should be over the limit then take the wheel.
And *nobody* should expect with status comes a deal.

SPECIAL BOY

So missed by all every single day.
Prayers for you every night I say.
Everyone misses your smiling face.
Called by Angels, Heaven to grace.
In dark times, memories rescue me.
All I could wish my little boy to be.
Lonely is my heart when days I cry.

Blue is the colour remembered by.
Our days of fun I relive and enjoy.
You'll forever be that 'special boy'

Let's Be Each Other

Do you fancy a swap, a barter or deal?
Maybe some arrangement we can seal.
Stole my space, do you want to be me?
Do you think I'm lucky as I park for free?

Do you crave a blue badge in your name?
Do you want to swap wellbeing for pain?
Maybe we should even go the whole way.
Let's be each other, and try that for a day.

Try my wheelchair for size, be my guest.
I can be you, with perfect health blessed.
You'll soon realise just how lucky you are.
And be glad that bay was meant for *my* car.

One Early Morn

Long ago in '77 a hero of mine.
Lost his life, he was just 29.
An unsafe car, results did find.
A 2 year old son he left behind.

He never learnt the driving skill.
But sang of cars and their thrill.
A life cut short of a star reborn.
As tragedy struck one early morn.

Many people have had their say.
On who was to blame for that day?
The driver survived that we know.
Did drink play a part, possibly so?

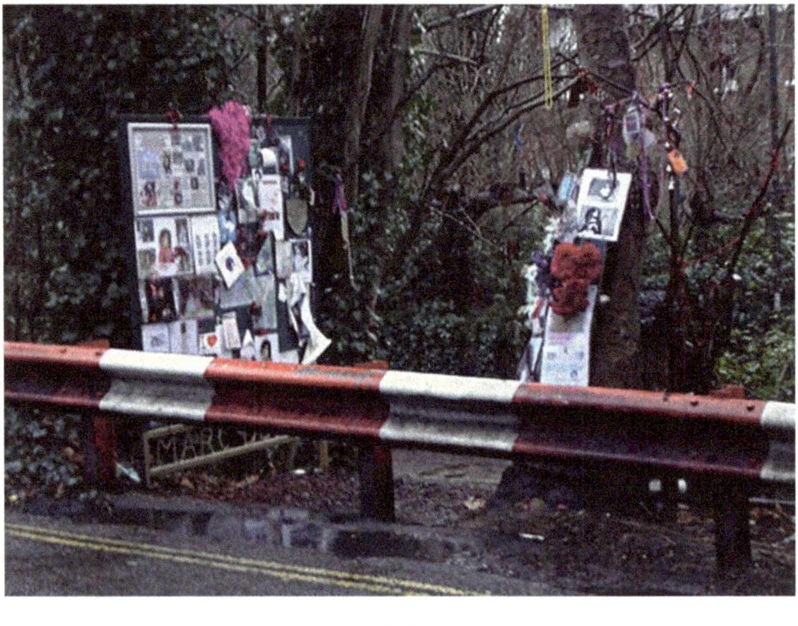

Pet Hate

We all have one, so what's your pet hate?
Drivers on roundabouts who don't indicate?
How about Taxi cabs who stop without care.
Anytime, anyplace when they spot a fare.

Cyclists on the road, who ride with no lights.
They can't be seen during dark winter nights.
Selfish motorists who park in disabled bays?
Drivers who litter in drive through take aways?

Overloaded cars with no rear window view.
Impatient drivers who speed to jump a queue.
Drivers who stop suddenly, confused or lost!
Rude fellow motorists, what do manners cost?

Think!

Think of the danger, consider the shame.
A day spent in Court, one tarnished name.
Money's no excuse for a cab not to call.
In both cases there's just no excuse at all.
And I don't care the colour of your shirt.
I care for other road users you could hurt.
Tragic outcomes I've seen time after time.
When selfish people commit such a crime.
If a hero to the young there's a role to play.
You've let everyone down driving that way.

Don't Hold Back

If a Bobby memory springs to mind.
Share it with me, it'll help you'll find.
And don't hold back in saying his name.
As to hear you say it, eases the pain.

If you're thinking back to days of fun.
All the daft things our kids have done!
If Bobby's part of those memories too.
Telling me might turn a dark sky blue.

If you're a blue, tell Bobby the score.
As Angels too can cheer and roar!
Keep Bobby in your thoughts every day.
Include him still when games you play.

If his name's on your lips, just let it go.
All your lovely memories I want to know.
Share them all with me, all of the time.
And I'll place them in this heart of mine.

Such memories help this heart to heal.
And they comfort me on lonely days I feel.
But on those days, God makes it known.
Bobby's only in Heaven, not far from home.

Gilles Vesco

A 'new mobilty' Vesco calls his vision and plan.
To rebalance public space between car and man.
A world with reduced noise and pollution far less.
A 'walkable city' for all with lack of vehicle stress.

Along Lyon's 2 rivers such change has took place.
The car parks where removed to create a space.
Human parks along those river banks now stand.
A pedestrian friendly area, a fairer use of the land.

Gilles Vesco uses a keyword, that word is 'share'
To produce a 'more walkable city' with cleaner air.
To rely less on the car might not appeal to some.
But the more attractive our cities will then become.

Cars stand idle for long periods, stats have shown.
Doing very little parked outside your work or home.
Car clubs, shared data with 'urban mobility' on call.
Improved public transport is the way forward for all.

Rail *Not* Road

In their lofty cabs sitting high.
Lorry drivers drive right by.
Stretching beyond legal lane.
Under pressure, time to gain.
Busy roads, a fight for space.
Too little room, creates a race.
With air pollution on the rise.
Diesel fumes make smoky skies.
I think of this as a system fail.
Free up the roads, turn to rail.
Driverless convoys soon to be.
Doesn't make any sense to me.
Share the burden and the weight.
Turn to rail, promote its freight.

HEARTBREAK

How long will this feeling remain?
Every sufferer must ask the same.
Actual bodily pain it feels for me.
Right now if I only could be free
To lose a young child in such a way.
Breaks my heart every single day.
Reminders, regrets, I have them all.
Every sad emotion has had its call.
All I want is a little less heartbreak
Kindness is my friend while I ache.

Michael Molloy

At a picture a Mum looks into a frame.
Michael Molloy, the young man's name.
5 years ago Michael never made it home.
Killed in a coach crash, an old tyre blown.

A 19 year old tyre, but not against the law.
3 lives innocent lives lost, tears to pour.
Old tyres often degrade from the inside.
The visible layers, the danger might hide.

But the law didn't seem to understand.
As such tyres on PSV's where not banned.
Join and support a Mums 'tyred' campaign.
Old tyres *did* kill, Michael Molly his name.

The New Generation

It's the way it is and the way it'll always be.
A generation moves on, a new one to see.
It's the way of the world, a good thing too.
The new generation, soon it's over to you!

Very eager no doubt with a point to prove.
Can't wait for 'old timers' to make a move!
Young blood at the ready to have their day.
To take on the world and to have their say!

When it comes to driving it's just the same.
So keen for lessons, a licence to your name.
But just take a step back and take on board.
Heed advice that should never be ignored.

Endless driving tips and hints you will hear.
Listen carefully, if not it might cost you dear.
Don't become impatient if setbacks you face.
Drive safe, show respect, that's a good base.

The most experienced driver will tell you so.
Something new will turn up, to learn or know.
Don't become complacent, continue to learn.
Keep all this mind when it becomes your turn.

Beat The Clock

I've seen it countless times before.
Impatience fuelled, pedal to the floor.
Other road users, they don't count.
Lanes to cross, pavements to mount.

Tolerance levels becoming very low.
Speeding to lights before red to glow.
Over speed bumps, sparks they fly.
Rev counters they soar into the high.

Dangerous drivers with a clock to beat.
A menace to us all on road and street.
Catch them and ban them every time.
Before tragedy becomes of their crime.

Less Afraid

What will I do with this brand new day?
File it under sadness and hide it away?
But plenty of friends who I can turn to.
Who will help me see this day through?

Always there for me, when feeling low.
People I love, hopefully I let it show.
Because on days that I can barely face.
It's hard to show love, not even a trace.

I need comfort most during such days.
When dark skies stifle all the Sun's rays.
That's when my friends come to my aid.
Their kindness makes me feel less afraid.

Melted Tears

I can feel it in my bones, feel it in the air.
All the signs are present; I am so aware.
Nothing I can do, nothing to put it right.
Just got to face it, a crying time tonight.
I can't bottle this up, no magic cap or lid.
Hopefully when I wake, all my tears be rid.
Maybe I'll be stronger for the day ahead.
As I will have no more tears left to shed.
And with dry eyes, I will take on the day.
Crying time over, God melted tears away.

Ghost Bike

Standing out in the gloom of night.
A small memorial, a sombre sight.
Standing still under lock and chain.
A cycle going nowhere in the rain.

Motionless wheels, pedals are still.
A reminder that cars can easily kill.
To be safe every cyclist has a right.
This is a 'Ghost Bike' painted white.

Tyres removed, stripped down frame.
Also known as 'whitecycle' by name.
Left in tribute at an 'accident' place.
A cyclist killed there in every case.

Eerie perhaps these bikes might be.
Something not everyone likes to see.
But just think on why they are there.
And show all cyclists respect and care.

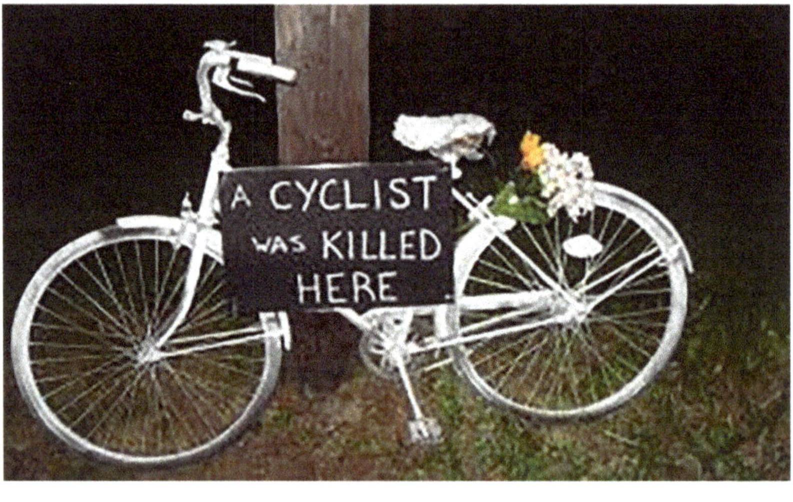

Self-Regulate

Just 2 years ago they introduced a new law.
To protect children's health it was meant for.
A new law that means well is all good by me.
Under 18's would ride in vehicles smoke free.

Now I'm not naive and I'm also not green!
My perfect world will still remain a pipe dream!
This new legislation, most will agree and say.
Will be impossible to enforce night and day.

So all responsible smokers should do the same.
'Self-regulation' being the name of the game.
Don't 'light up' with children in the front *or* back.
While driving just hide away that cigarette pack.

In Bed By 8!

Disabled drivers *do* shop when it's dark.
So remember that before you illegally park.
Or are you the type that just couldn't care?
Long as you're happy, you park anywhere.

Many drivers abuse disabled bays at night.
In fast food stores it's such a common sight.
The usual suspects and culprits there to see.
Stealing a blue badge bay in a midnight KFC.

I know what they'll think in their tiny mind.
No disabled drivers at midnight they will find.
They don't go out at midnight to eat and drink.
That's what these selfish idiots probably think.

It goes on in leisure centre too, once it's late.
Blue badge holders probably in bed by eight!
That must be these offenders train of thought.
It won't stop until they're punished and caught.

Gone Tomorrow

I hate this feeling, stuck like glue.
All hemmed in a huge traffic queue.
Crawling traffic to my left and right.
Feel suffocated when space is tight.

It stretches miles ahead and behind.
No escape route is ever easy to find.
Bumper to bumper, in the warm sun.
A nightmare journey this has become.

Tangible frustration I sense all around.
I want to feel my feet on the ground.
Offer me reliable, cheaper bus or rail.
My car be gone tomorrow without fail.

Running Late

Running late, it's happened to us all.
Slept right through an alarm clock call!
Breakfast rushed, your head in a spin!
The first school lesson already kicked in.

Mind unclear, you can't think straight.
You hate the fact that you'll be late.
Chill out, relax, call the school to explain.
Don't be rushing to catch a bus or train.

That's how accidents happen you know.
When your concentration levels are low.
'Better late than ever' is always the case.
Road safety comes first over time to race.

Aftermaths

You know in this country what we say.
4 seasons of weather in just one day!
Autumn, Summer, Winter and Spring.
Different emotions each one can bring.

But there's an emotion never to change.
It doesn't care what the weather range.
The emotion of heartache, such as mine.
Though I might try to hide it time to time.

It comes back stronger with added guilt.
It's like it won't allow my life to be rebuilt.
Aftermaths of a road death run and run.
Especially if the loss, was your young son.

Vulnerable Still

Don't think you're invincible if a helmet you wear.
Stats show cars give you even less room to spare.
A crash helmet *will* get you out of the odd scrape.
But from the full force of a car, there's little escape.
We all understand 'prevention is better than cure'
So improve your cycling skills, ride within the law.
And if you're a parent teaching your children to ride.
Helmets give confidence as with pads to knees tied.
But there is no substitute in learning the correct skill.
As *all* cyclists with helmets remain so vulnerable still.

Monsters In A Cage

Its rush hour, peak hour, road traffic overkill.
Frustrated, fed up, drivers, patience levels nil.
Now once placid people, monsters in a cage.
Welcome to societies, modern day road rage

Anger all around, motorists personal little war.
Every inch of space, seems worth fighting for.
Fists, I see them waving, the air is turning blue.
Some lane hopper, has jumped a traffic queue!

Noise levels rising, wispy fumes pollute the air.
Bored looking passengers from a window stare.
I couldn't drive through that every working day.
If you have the choice, maybe find another way.

More Than Ever

And a 'Merry Christmas' to you too!
What an inconsiderate thing to do.
'A busy time of year' I hear you say.
Pressies to buy, Santa's on his way!

In a mad dash and deadlines to beat.
It's been 'all go' rushed of your feet.
If that's all true, you've still no right.
To steal what's mine, day and night,

And think this before you steal my bay.
The disabled also have Christmas Day.
The same hectic schedule we also face.
So more than ever we need that space.

NEAR TO SCHOOL

Near to a school at finishing time.
Enter the area, obey every sign.
At all times be alert, be aware.
Roads are there for all to share.

Turn your lights on, be easy to see.
Only park where supposed to be.

Slow right down, even to a crawl.
Caution all around, children small.
Hazard and perception be the rule.
On lookout for danger by a school.
Our kids are precious, so drive slow.
Lead by example is the way to go!

RoadPeace Wood

At RoadPeace wood, a special place I see.
Living and growing tributes in every tree.
Grown in tribute of loved ones taken away.
A place to reflect, to remember or to pray.
Somewhere to gather, memories to share.
To lean on a shoulder, to show you care.
Sponsor a tree, a few loving words to say.
To be seen by future generations every day.
An evolving, uplifting remembrance place.
Where nature and emotion come face to face.

Dark Is The Hour

Dark is the hour on this Autumn night.
I will think of my Angel until daylight.
I will search for answers, I will not sleep.
Sorrows pain tonight attacks me deep.

I'll need God's help tomorrow for sure.
If only for heartache there was a cure.
3 years on I miss him more by the day.
All my love sent to Heaven is on its way.

Maybe when he gets it, he'll send a sign.
The kind my Angel sends me time to time.
Those signs remain forever in my heart.
And only in the flesh do we remain apart.

Daybreak now, I see clouds low and grey.
Strength is mine, God has sent it my way.
With that strength, I will see this through.
But tears will still flow, as they always do.

Snippets

Snippets of my past sometimes come to me
Because of a place or music or some old TV.
They *can* be an intrusion, my heart to steal.
It depends on my state of mind on how I feel.

But at times they are welcome I have to say.
Those snippets pick me up on a lonely old day.
I know I can't control them, so what can I do?
Mostly I love them as they remind me of you.

But other times they hurt me and make me sad.
Because then I miss the best times I ever had.
If a reckless driver long ago didn't race or speed.
Then these words about snippets I wouldn't need.

Avoidable Vehicle Breakdown

This is something you may not know.
If you run out of fuel and need a tow.
In certain areas an FPN you could face.
So don't let it happen in the first place.

Avoidable breakdowns are on the rise.
Fluids not topped up or a battery dies.
Before long journeys take time and care.
Are your tyres legal, including the spare?

Check all fluid levels, water, oil and so.
Don't wait for that warning light to glow.
Such breakdowns can be dangerous too.
So make sure they never happen to you.

An Unnatural Death

An unnatural death, no last goodbye.
And over and over, I ask myself why?
Why are many lives lost in this way?
An unacceptable stat, 4,000 each day.

Violent road deaths, carnage untold.
One tragedy after another to unfold.
This shouldn't be allowed to carry on.
Let's make change, make this day one

Follow RoadPeace, be part of our plan.
Help fight our cause, however you can.
This death and destruction has to stop.
The figures for road deaths *have* to drop.

Stolen Summers

Now three years ago, one terribly sad day.
God invited a young boy to Heaven to play.
That didn't make sense and it made us cry.
I suppose only God knows the reason why.

Life's rules where broken for a young Mum.
Should I not see the growing up of my son?
Deprived of my boy, replaced with this pain.
Every Summer stolen and replaced with rain.

Time drags today, every minute like an hour.
I shed a tear with every poem, every flower.
I look at Bobby's tree, one big symbol of love.
While I look up for strength to Heaven above.

'Thrill Seekers'

Risking harm to others for kicks to achieve.
Riding into busy traffic, in and out to weave.
Leaving themselves with little time to brake.
They're putting all road users' life's at stake.
These 'dare devil' cyclists one day could kill.
All in pursuit of danger, to seek a road thrill.
No point or purpose I see in this biking craze.
Exhilarate yourselves in less dangerous ways.
Road traffic laws should move with the times.
To charge these offenders with road crimes.

3 Reasons Why

Before you board your car, engine to ignite.
Is it a lovely day, weather warm and bright?
Will your car journey be long, travelling far?
If not, are you simply too reliant on your car?

Are you about the tackle a busy school run?
Is it too far to walk when all said and done?
Are you friends or neighbours going that way?
Why not share your car, take turns each day?

Is public transport available, take a bus ride?
You'll also have the environment on your side!
Change your habits occasionally, give it a try.
Healthier, cheaper, less stress 3 reasons why!

Feeling Blessed

I see a little Robin looking down at me.
He's playing hide and seek from a tree.
And he's took away that November rain.
And just like last time, eased my pain.

Thank you Robin, my Robin red breast.
The sun now shines, I'm feeling blessed.
I know it's a sign when all said and done.
See you next time, my loving little son.

Farewell as you take to the now blue sky.
I know this won't be our last Goodbye.
Sit on the roses next time, rest your wings.
And let me hear how a little Angel sings.

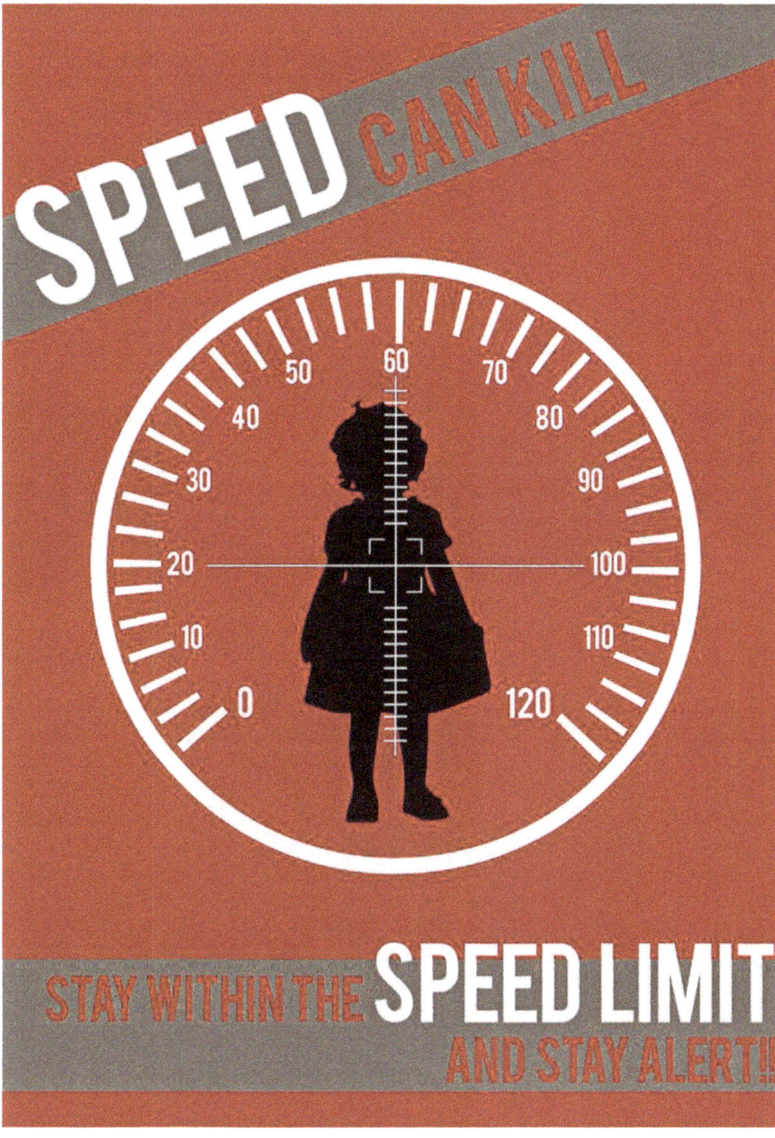
SPEED CAN KILL
50
60
70
40
80
30
90
20
100
10
110
0
120
STAY WITHIN THE SPEED LIMIT
AND STAY ALERT!!

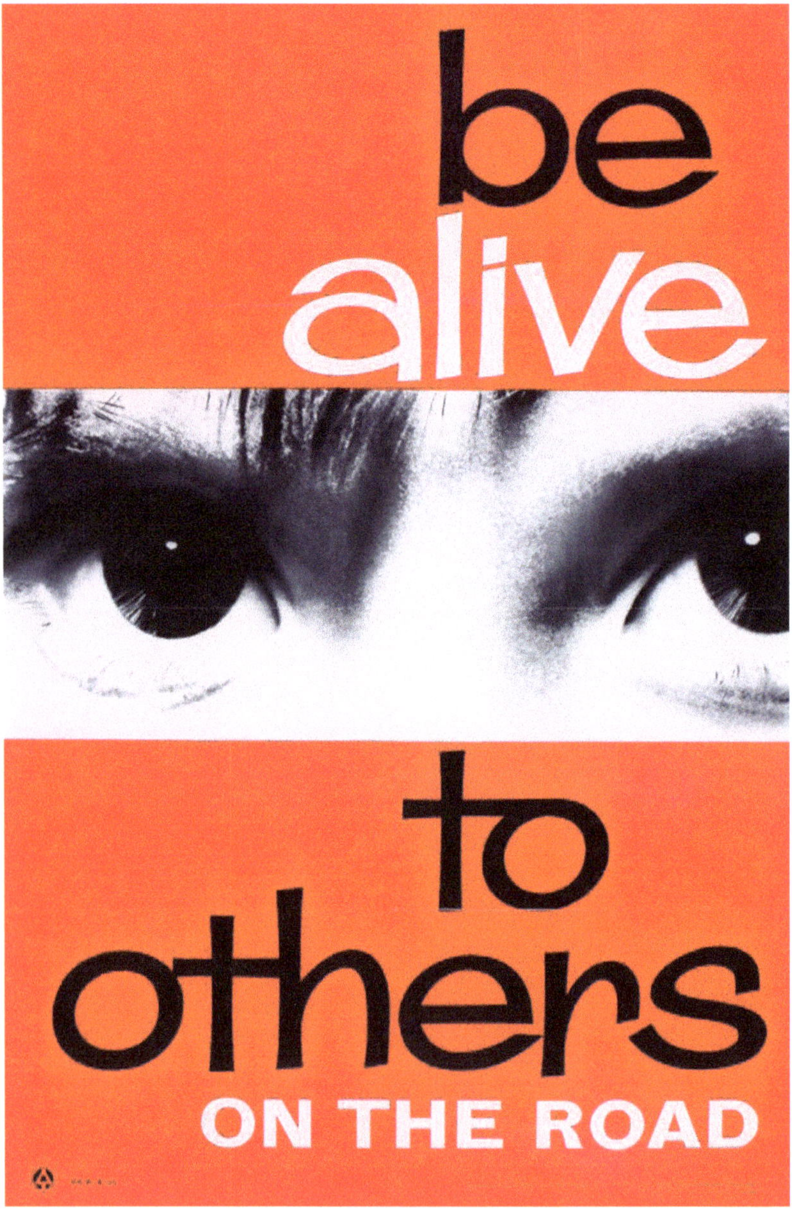
be
alive
to
others
ON THE ROAD

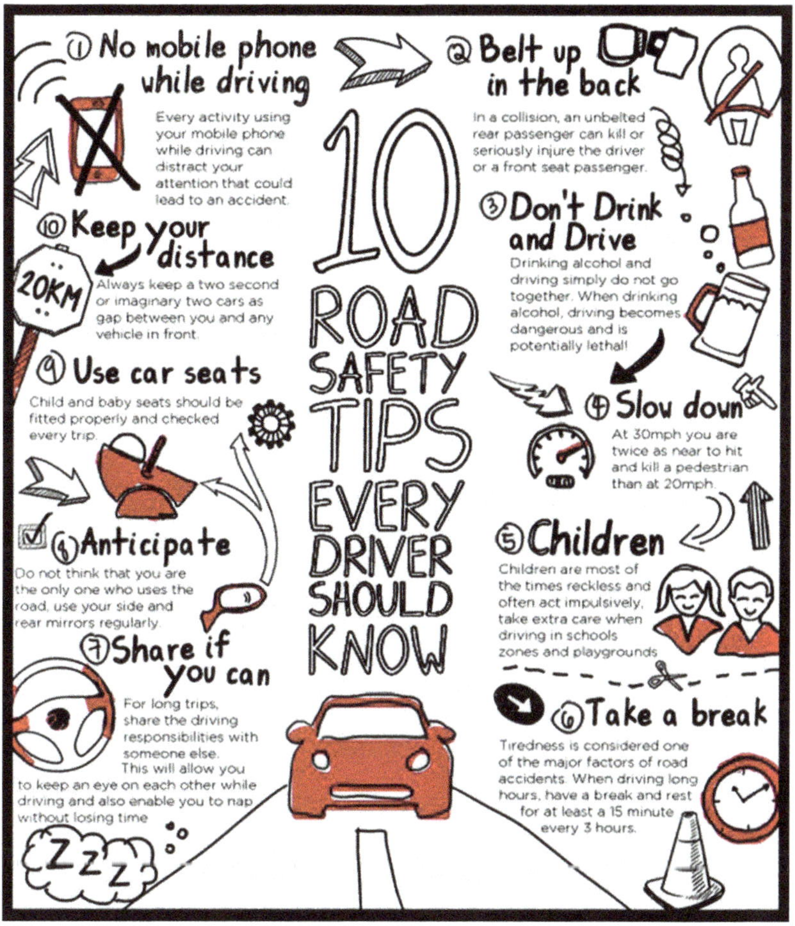

10 ROAD SAFETY TIPS EVERY DRIVER SHOULD KNOW
① No mobile phone while driving
Every activity using your mobile phone while driving can distract your attention that could lead to an accident.
② Belt up in the back
In a collision, an unbelted rear passenger can kill or seriously injure the driver or a front seat passenger.
③ Don't Drink and Drive
Drinking alcohol and driving simply do not go together. When drinking alcohol, driving becomes dangerous and is potentially lethal!
④ Slow down
At 30mph you are twice as near to hit and kill a pedestrian than at 20mph.
⑤ Children
Children are most of the times reckless and often act impulsively, take extra care when driving in schools zones and playgrounds
⑥ Take a break
Tiredness is considered one of the major factors of road accidents. When driving long hours, have a break and rest for at least a 15 minute every 3 hours.
⑦ Share if you can
For long trips, share the driving responsibilities with someone else. This will allow you to keep an eye on each other while driving and also enable you to nap without losing time
⑧ Anticipate
Do not think that you are the only one who uses the road, use your side and rear mirrors regularly.
⑨ Use car seats
Child and baby seats should be fitted properly and checked every trip.
⑩ Keep your distance
Always keep a two second or imaginary two cars as gap between you and any vehicle in front.
20KM
ZZZ

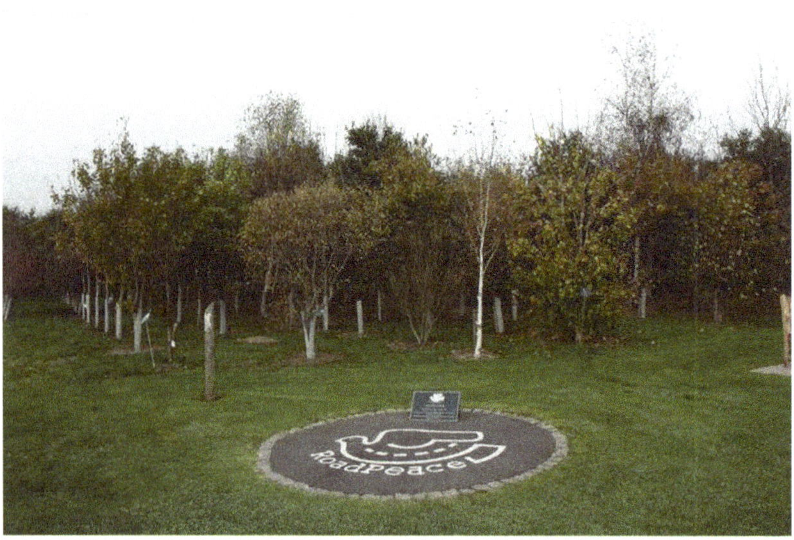
RoadPeace

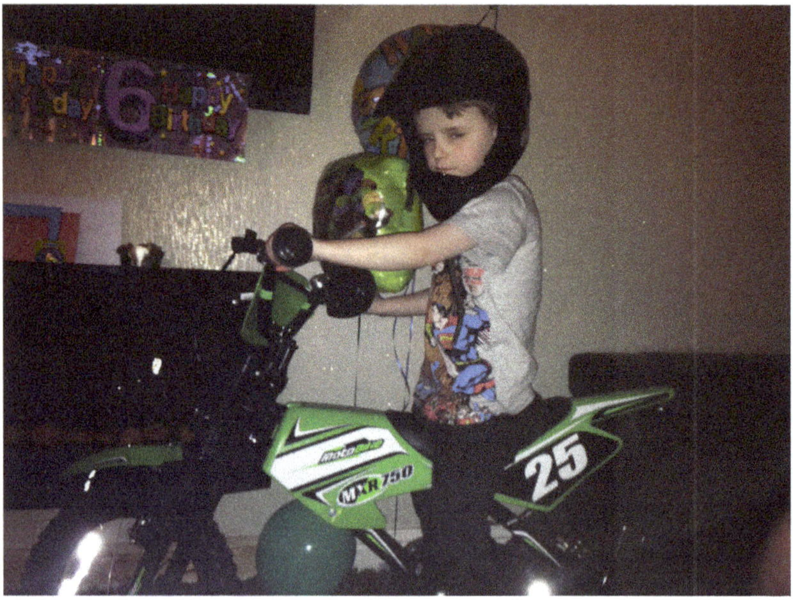
MXR 750
25

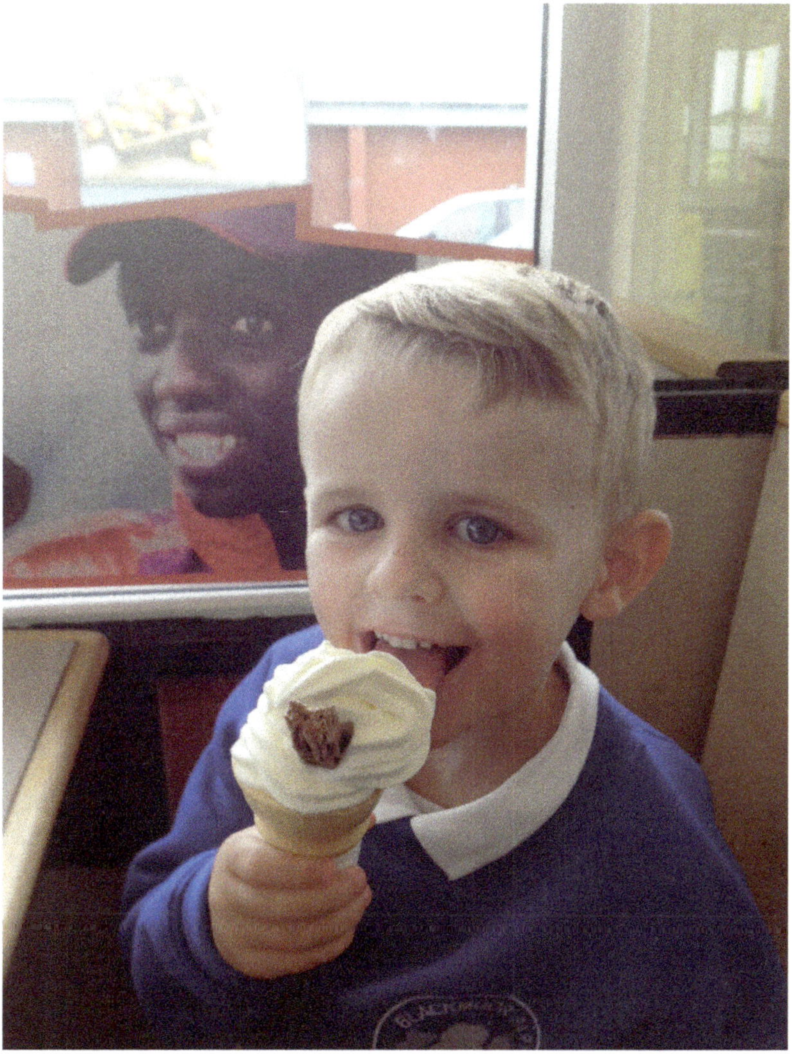

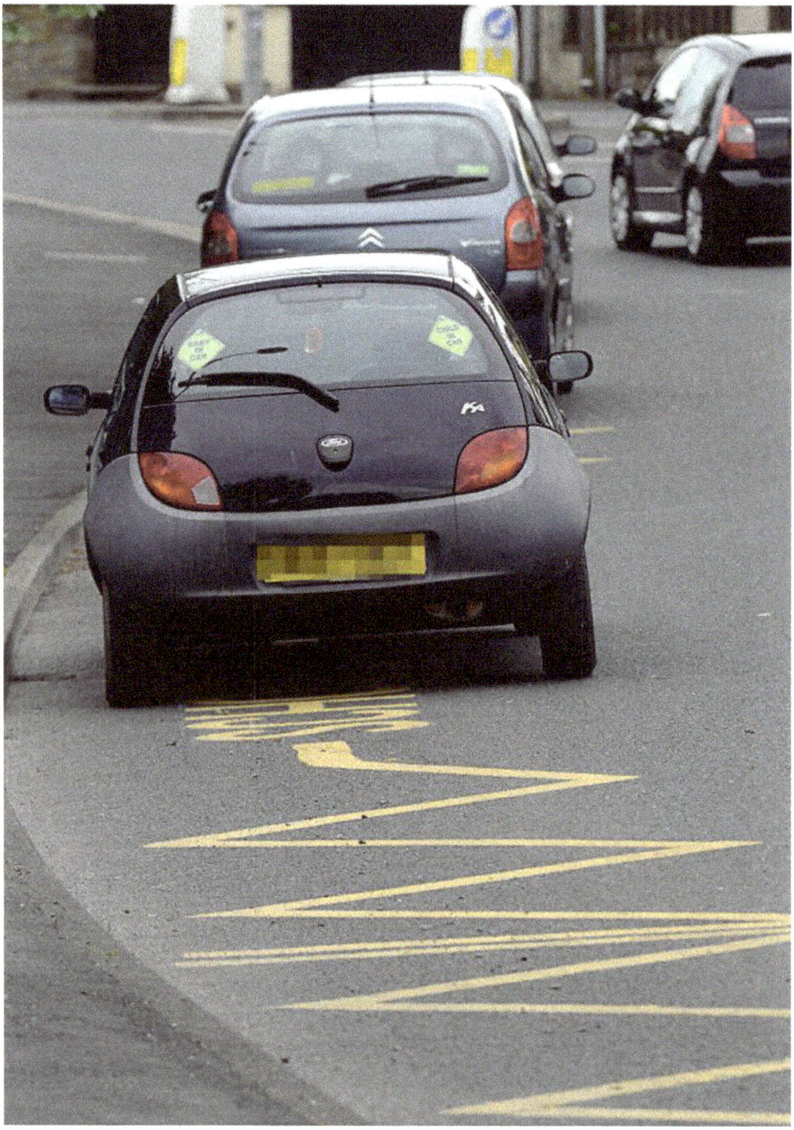

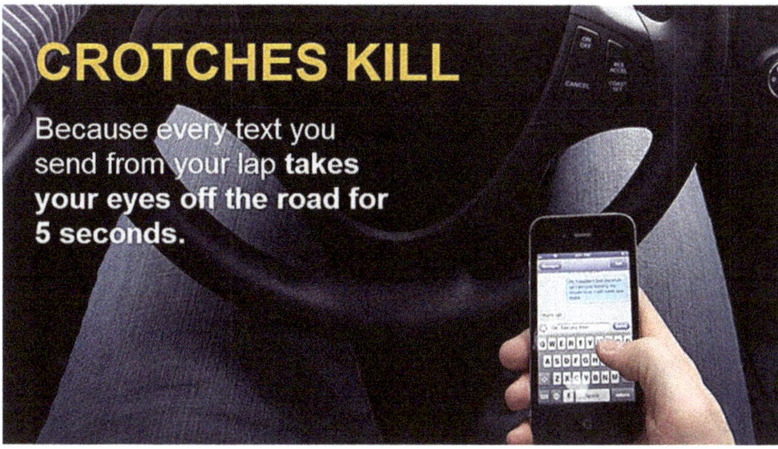
CROTCHES KILL
Because every text you send from your lap **takes your eyes off the road for 5 seconds.**

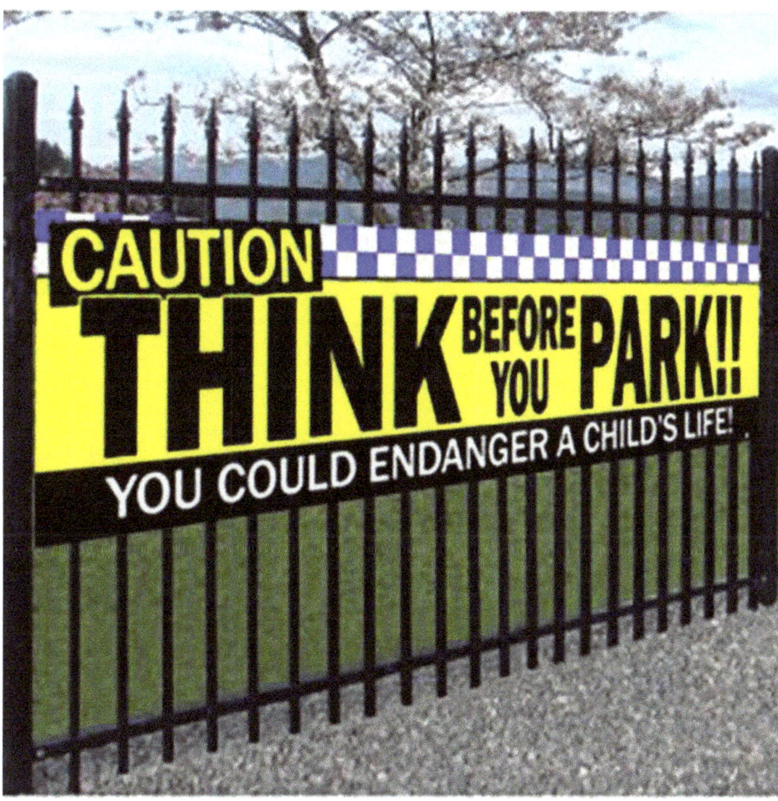
CAUTION
THINK BEFORE YOU PARK!!
YOU COULD ENDANGER A CHILD'S LIFE!

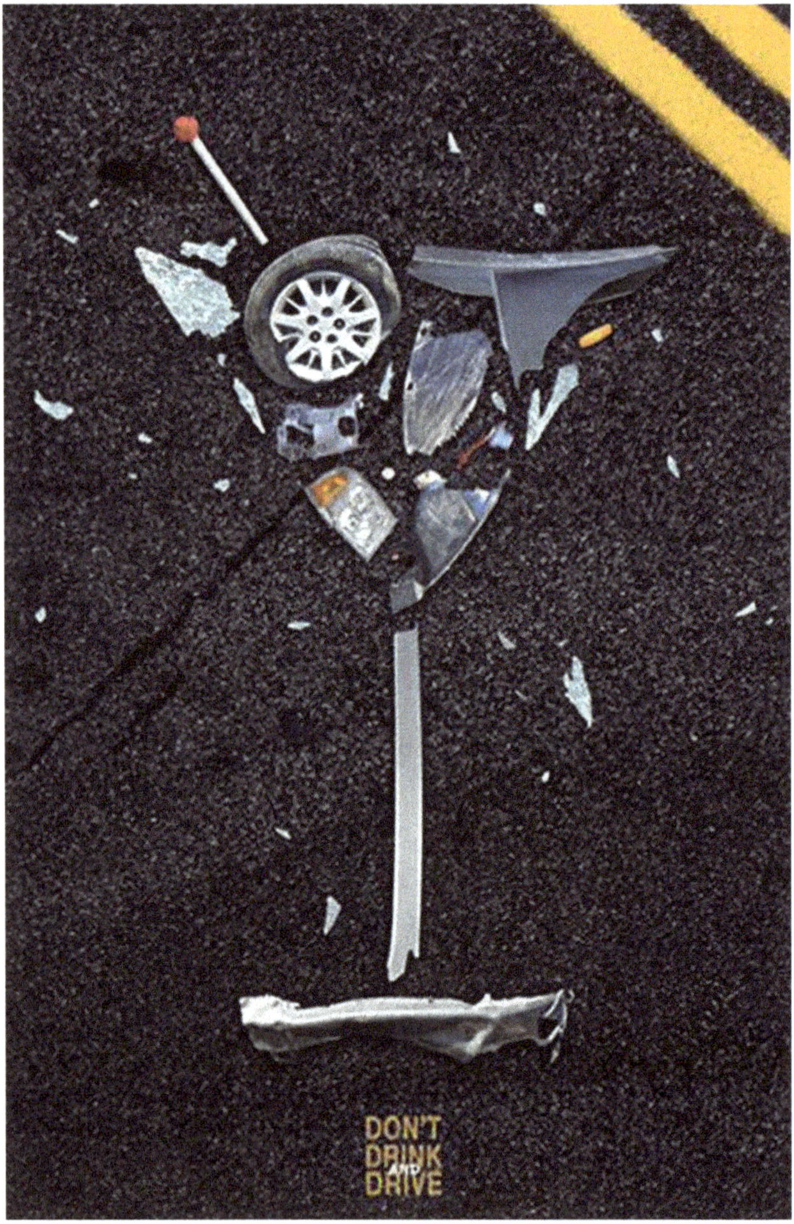
DON'T
DRINK
AND
DRIVE

Dangerous Brew

Am I out being of order, is it just me?
Am I being judgemental in what I see?
It's just my opinion, can't claim it fact.
Do certain cars, selfish drivers attract?

I mean top of the range Audi and so.
And 4x4's that have never seen snow.
All image and speed a dangerous brew.
Is it just me, or do you think its true?

One thing for sure, as I see it every day.
I see plenty such cars in a disabled bay.
No blue badge do all those drivers hold.
Lazy, ignorant people who can't be told.

SPEED KILLS

Speeding drivers, a danger in every way.
Putting innocent lives at risk every day
Every MPH is vital should a collision occur.
Every driver of that fact should be aware.
Don't cause devastation, untold heartache.

Keep well within the limit, no risks to take.
In built up areas, speed must be kept low.
Lives will be needlessly lost if that's not so.
Lost control through speed, easy you'll find.
Speed kills, that's a fact, keep that in mind.

Beer Goggles

Put the beer goggles on, go for a ride.
Tackle a test drive with 6 pints inside.
It's an upside world, vision like a bee.
Vision impaired, you'll struggle to see.

You're driving from just memory alone.
And you can't make out corner or cone.
Judgement impaired, control at a loss.
Problem after problem you come across.

All but disappeared has your driving skill.
On real life roads you might injure and kill.
Don't let that happen, stop first and think.
Never mix driving with too much to drink.

When Breezes Come

When breezes come and make branches shake.
When the snow leans on twigs until they break.
The colourful decorations will still shine through.
Because this tree is special, Robins think so too!

Other trees in the world maybe steeped in fame.
The Hardy Tree and The Hyperion just 2 to name
The Major Oak, in which Robin Hood would hide.
The Sunland Baobab, which has a little bar inside!

The General Sherman Tree reaches into the sky.
All such trees are famous, for good reasons why.
But none can boast a Robin who visits time to time.
And none have to Bobby a 'Merry Christmas' sign.

Not Long Ago

I long for those days, not long ago.
When rain was rain, snow was snow.
Problems solved with such ease.
Swept aside in the Autumn breeze.

I long for those days, not long ago.
When yes meant yes, no meant no.
These days now I seem so unsure.
Nothing makes much sense anymore.

I long for those days, not long ago.
When dirty faces still would glow.
Straight forward was the World to me.
Now one and one seem to make three.

I long for those days, not long ago.
Before I knew hearts could sink so low.
But in Gods time I know I'll get there.
Just stand close by me, show you care.

The Sky Wore Blue

Did you see the Liverpool sky today?
All grey clouds where banished away.
Nothing up there for rainbows to chase.
Spring at long last had shown its face.
No March snow fall under skies of white.
The sun it shone, so warm and bright.
Who knows what tomorrow might bring.
Will Winter return in place of Spring?
But today to Spring the weather was true.
As for Bobby today, the sky wore blue.

Driving With Dementia

A driver in denial of mental health decline.
She ignored every increasing warning sign.
Stall after stall, clutch control on the wane.
The reassuring answer, the car to blame.

Roundabouts became a nightmarish sight.
Taking multiple attempts to get an exit right.
Unable to judge corners or a simple bend.
Keeping a straight line, a struggle in the end.

No accidents she caused only through luck.
One day a tragedy would have likely struck.
Before that day had a chance to take place.
She confronted her denial with reality to face.

She gave up her licence in line with the law.
A brave decision she could no longer ignore.
Advice from friends and family she listened to.
Please do the same if dementia's affecting you.

Rise of The Parking Vigilante

It's reported on social media more and more.
It makes people's anger levels soar and soar.
Selfish, inconsiderate parking, it's on the rise.
Naming and shaming offenders is no surprise.

It's happening all over, sites popping up online.
Some people don't approve, but to me it's fine.
These selfish drivers who openly flout the law.
Who mustn't care what a school crossing is for.

They park where they could block a child's view.
If a danger to children, I would shame them too.
Narrow pavements are not for vehicles to share.
But selfish, ignorant drivers obviously don't care.

Stronger Deterrent

It didn't take long into my walk today.
Till I saw a mobile user chatting away.
Driving along, one hand on the wheel.
An innocent life, today he might steal.

It beggars belief it still widely goes on.
Show me a good reason, there is none.
For some drivers is the legality a blur?
Yet some offenders probably don't care.

Male, female drivers, across the board.
Paltry fine if caught, too easy to afford.
And even when a fine *is* hefty and steep.
It matters little when pockets run deep.

And a licence endorsed, again big deal.
Often waived after a rich man's appeal.
An instant driving ban is the way to go.
A stronger deterrent they have to show.

Skies of Grey

When a live needs to be rebuilt.
Happiness may come with guilt.
And even with a sense of shame.
For letting go of some deep pain.

This is natural as human we are.
We bear the brunt of every scar.
The healing process to our heart.
Unexpectedly one day will start.

Departed souls to be loved no less.
Every day still to cherish and bless.
The miracle of life has this way.
To see us through all skies of grey.

A 'Cars Width'

No wonder poor cyclists get annoyed.
Stuck in the gutter, potholes to avoid.
Or pools of water, from flooded drain.
It *can* be a tricky and dangerous terrain.
So if you approach a cyclist to overtake.
Be cautious and take care for their sake.
Treat cycles like another car on the road.
Heed the advice from the Highway Code.
Please afford cycles a 'car widths' space.
In case they *have* to pull out and at pace.

One For The Superhero

I look to the Sky and see a bike of green.
A flowing red cape in the sun does gleam.
He rides the skies on two wheels I see.
I can't make him out, who could this be?

Superman is one of many heroes of mine.
But I don't think its 'Supie' not this time.
Maybe it's Batman, the caped crusader?
Or is he an alien, a kind of space invader?

Now I see him riding down from the skies.
That cheeky grin no costume can disguise!
Its SuperBob, and if luck be on your side.
By your school you might just see SB ride!

And if you do see him, don't forget to wave.
If you're by a road, watch how you behave!
Because although SB is watching out for you.
Children have a part to play in road safety too.

At crossings wait for the green man to show.
Then still look both ways, until it's safe to go.
Then you'll make SuperBob happy and smile.
Before he rides away to the skies for a while.

Who is the greatest Superhero, no need to ask!
The road safety guardian, ready for every task.
And if SuperBob has seen how clever you are.
You will shine as bright as a silver Sheriff star!

You can tell all your friends and Mum and Dad.
That you saw a Superhero, and made him glad.
And all your family will be happy, you will see.
Because you showed how sensible you can be!

Just Another Cheat

The time of day to do a 'big shop'
Blue Badge on display, out I pop.
I eventually find a disabled bay.
Some people seem to mutter away.

They're not convinced at all by me.
They're right, I'm healthy as can be.
I do my shopping, its takes a while.
Something needed from every aisle.

I chat to friends, they ask, they care.
They ask about Mum, her wheelchair.
As they see me alone in the queue.
They ask has she come shopping too.

I tell them no, I prefer to shop alone.
Her wheelchair is best left at home.
I return to my car, just another cheat.
But thankfully no wardens on the beat.

To abuse the blue badge in that vein.
Is fraudulent misuse, no other name.
Its laziness, its illegal, it's another case.
Of thieving a disabled parking space.

The Chain

Cause a road death, you start a chain.
And with every link, will travel the pain.
Family and friends, the first tears to flow.
Work and school mates, teachers like so.
When I pass such sites like 'Bobby's Tree'
Also the wider community it seems to me.
All down the line there's further heartache.
And like any chain, it's so difficult to break.
So drive within the law, no chain to create.
Change your ways today, before it's too late.

Life Time Ban

Look in your car mirror, when you speed.
Do you see a person with an ego to feed?
Maybe your self-esteem is in short supply.
So does braking the law, make it feel high?

Speeding drivers baffle me, they really do.
If out to impress, the very opposite is true.
They're just a selfish, low life waste of space.
And on our busy roads, they have no place.

And those with a long history of this offence.
A life time driving ban, makes perfect sense.
Their actions might cause a fatality one day.
So ban them for good, take that chance away.

Photograph

I wonder how this day will go.
Impossible anymore to know.
Then I look at a picture of old.
Now I know how it will unfold.

A beautiful pic 4 years gone.
Today, a day *not* to 'move on'
How can I, impossible for me.
Just look exactly at what I see.

This picture today that I share.
Breaks my heart beyond repair.
Today I cry, I reflect and I pine.
Moving on…is for another time

Roundabouts

A simple way to help traffic flow free.
Though not every drivers cup of tea.
Uncertainty at times I see all around.
Car horns blasting, a common sound.

They're cheap to install and to maintain.
And they're not too taxing on the brain.
But so many drivers pull out or weave.
And never signal when an exit to leave.

But these circular roads when used right.
I think work just as well as a traffic light.
The good old Roundabout hated by some.
But used correctly they get the job done.

October

The month of October, the 10th of the calendar year.
Shops want you thinking that Christmas time is near!
The month rounded off, by Halloween's trick or treat.
Children in scary costumes, up and down your street.

An Autumn month, with fine weather mixed with rain.
An emotional time for me, in the shape of added pain.
Towards the end of October, fireworks light up the sky.
But it's a month that I hope just quickly passes me by.

As my little boy was taken away, one sad October day.
If only it was possible, to simply wish this month away.
It used to be a special month, I so looked forward too.
But now I want it gone, disappear like the morning dew.

DEVASTATED

Dismayed at the road death of my son.
Endless hurdles faced to get justice done.
Valid concerns for a system out of date.
Appalled the police failed to investigate.
Sympathy and advice, little given to me.
The apathy of our politicians plain to see.
An 'accident' was clearly the wrong term.
The powers that be have so much to learn.
Every 'preventable collision' is a real crime.
Dismayed at leniency shown time after time.

The Bobmobile!

Now that's what I call a special car!
A vehicle that stands out from a far.
Special words we all need to share.
They can even be seen from the air!
And of those words please take note.
Road safety for kids, please promote.
Read the fantastic books all about 'SB'
Support Bobby's trust, visit the tree.
Move over Batmobile, this is my fave!
If you see this car, please give a wave!

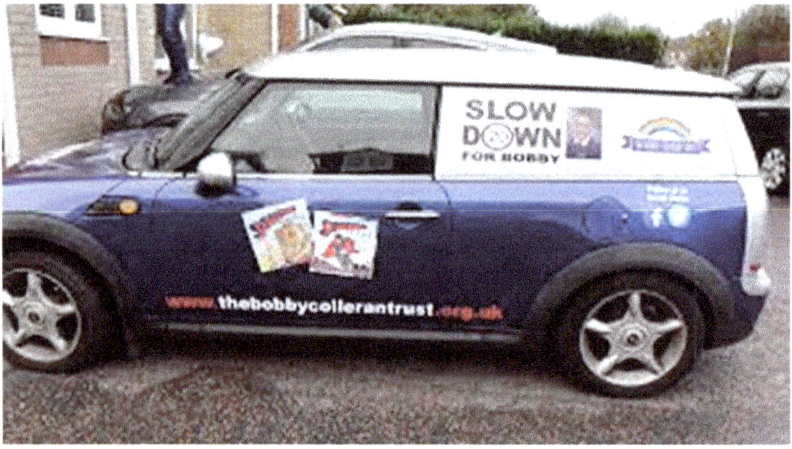

Disabled Parking Bay Thieves

You see it in Supermarkets every day.
Lazy drivers parking in a disabled bay.
You know the type, cocky and brash.
Jumping out of the car, quick as a flash.

A 'hidden disability' I hardly think so?
I don't see a disabled badge on show.
Some shops don't care and never will.
As long as their money rings in the till.

Such people must be devoid of all pride.
No shame taking the system for a ride.
So happy I wasn't dragged up that way.
Respect only themselves, is what I say.

But have a word with them face to face.
Ask why they take up a disabled space.
Normally you get verbal abuse in return.
When will these selfish people ever learn?

The Rock

You sit close beside me when I cry.
You have an answer when I ask why.
On your shoulder I can always lean.
Tell me reasons I still have to dream.
If I lose control, you're always there.
Guiding me through days of despair.
You pick up the pieces of my heart.
How do I thank you, where to start?
You're there for me around the clock.
Where would I be, without my rock?

Where's The Glamour?

Speeding glamourised in movies, on TV.
It sends out the wrong messages to me.
Leading to dangerous boundaries to push.
Encouraging a motoring adrenaline rush.

So many modern day cars built for speed.
With restricted speed limits, I see no need?
In television land it's probably safe to say.
There's not much risk testing cars that way.

It's those copycat drivers I'm afraid to find.
Whose only aim is to leave the rest behind.
On our everyday busy roads, it goes on still.
Where's the glamour, after these driver's kill?

Golden Rule

A group of children by the school gate.
The last lesson over, no longer to wait!
Family and friends to hurry and greet.
Facebook to activate and stuff to tweet!

And that moment can't come too soon.
To hear once more your favourite tune!
It seems like forever, but it's just a day.
So ear phones then worn to hear it play!

Does this type of behaviour apply to you?
If so, can you think for a moment or two?
And will you do a little favour just for me?
As another tragedy we don't want to see.

When by those gates outside your school.
Think of your road safety, the golden rule.
Don't be distracted, let fun and games wait.
That golden rule is, to please concentrate.

At an early age children should be taught.
That *all* roads with danger can be fraught.
But as they get older, this is also my view.
Children have to be more responsible too.

The Rich and Famous

How many times has it happened before?
The rich and famous seem above the law.
Lenient punishments for their road crime.
Millionaires are 'punished' with a paltry fine.

Be it sports star, person of stage or screen.
It appears like 'them and us' no in between.
They hire the best defence money can buy.
A 'classless society' I hear, I don't see why.

Let's not forget pop stars and politicians too.
I think different rules apply to me and you.
In one case a ban for speeding not applied.
Caught well over the limit, luckily nobody died.

3 past speeding offences already to his name.
The Judge fell for his excuses, all of them lame.
A famous politician crashed, mobile in hand.
6 points reduced to 3, to save getting banned.

I'm one of the 'great unwashed' and proud to be.
For similar crimes they'd throw the book at me.
Anyone guilty of road crime, whoever the case.
Should expect the same heavy punishment to face.

Consideration

Be considerate, the road is to share.
Look out for cyclists, respect and care.
At many traffic lights there is a space.
This box is for cyclists, it's there place.

It give them time to pull away on green.
A protection measure in a traffic stream.
A safety zone countless drivers ignore.
To encroach this area is against the law.

It's selfish behaviour behind the wheel.
All for a few metres and seconds to steal.
But cyclists have to be considerate too.
I see many at red lights riding on through.

One Minute For Bobby

I just have these few words to say.
Please put a minute aside today.
So many minutes in a day to spend.
Put one away, just the one to lend.

Stop what you're doing if it can wait.
So what, if something trivial is late.
Most people have 1 minute to spare.
Just sixty seconds to show you care.

Turn off your computer, phone or TV.
From a hectic world set yourself free.
Think of young Bobby, his cheeky grin!
And let that one minute belong to him.

3 years ago today young Bobby died.
Killed on our roads, as one we cried.
A life needlessly cut short on that day.
Through tears our respects now we pay.

A HIT AND RUN

An act so cowardly, such an immoral thing to do.

How do you look in the mirror if it applies to you?
Inside, how do you live with the guilt and shame?
To cause death or injury but to shoulder no blame.

And what kind of souls do such people possess?
Not thinking of their victims, their pain or distress.
Driving on regardless, the scene to escape or flee.

Refusing aid and attention, the saddest part to me.
Unconcerned of their actions, just an escape to find.
No worry of the tragedy they might have left behind.

Why?

Why is a crime not considered a *real* crime?
Why are corners cut to save money and time?
And why is a 'violet death' is not considered so.
All these things the bereaved need to know.
Why aren't past convictions taken into account?
Why are families given hurdles to mount?
Why are most jail sentences frustratingly light?
Why for justice and peace do we have to fight?
Why is help and support in such short supply?
Like so many others, I can only ask myself why.

No Interest

Aggressive young drivers, angry and rude.
They only seem to know one driving mood.
But they 'own the road' don't you know?
Impatient to all drivers *they* think are slow.

Right pedal normally rammed to the floor.
Consider themselves above the driving law.
Flash people, flash cars, exhausts a plenty.
Can be seen doing 30, when signs say 20.

Do such drivers care, I think not one bit?
An unnatural death for those they might hit.
They have no interest in our RoadPeace call.
These drivers are a major danger to us all.

Keep Those Robins Flying

Please little Bobby, keep those Robins flying.
Landing close beside me, comfort any crying.
I know from Heaven, those Robins are a sign.
Every visit is special and cheer me every time.

They have come to greet me and to say 'hello'
You're a happy boy, their presence tells me so.
You are safe in Gods care, every day and night.
A Robin lets me know this when within my sight.

So when I see a Robin, with red upon his breast.
I'm reassured my little Angel is peacefully at rest.
So keep those Robins flying, tears they will dry.
Keep watching over me, from up there in the sky.

.

The School Run Chore

Fancy a bit more walking and driving less?
You'll save some money and feel less stress!
Stop start, parking pain, on the school run.
That's not what I call common sense or fun!
If you don't live far from school give it a trial.
Just make some effort to walk once a while.
Unstrap your children from their car seat.
Let them feel fresh air and exercise their feet.
That's far more fun than stuck in a traffic line.
Turn the school run chore into quality time!

The Traffic Memorial

A bronze Teddy bear rests at its base.
A little child's doll looks forlorn in face.
Sitting in all weathers, patiently to wait.
A doll who's missing her little playmate.

I see a victim's discarded walking cane.
Another life lost, another buried name.
2 fingers on a wrist watch frozen in time.
A set of keys lie beside this 'traffic sign'

A ladies handbag, a fallen mobile phone.
Items of victims who never made it home.
A moving inscription, in words very few.
Lives unfulfilled, in every case sadly true.

If you visit Liverpool, even just for a day.
Go to St Johns Gardens during your stay.
Visit this sculpture, put one moment aside.
Respect every victim who needlessly died.

Pavement Parking

Sketchy UK laws make it unclear across the land.
In London pavement parking is simply banned.
In Exeter and in Worcester applies the same law.
But in the rest of the Country, we're a bit unsure.

Either way, it's a problem increasing by the day.
Vehicles parking on busy a pavement or walkway.
A sign 'should not' park might be seen time to time.
This is largely ignored without fear of ticket or fine.

Because local authorities tend to turn a blind eye.
Expensive, time consuming red tape the reason why.
Charities Living Street and Guide Dog lead the way.
They want such parking punished all over the UK.

This type of parking can be such a danger to some.
Blocked paths for the visually impaired can't be fun.
And parents with prams should expect a clear route.
The pavement is for pedestrians, not drivers to suit.

London's pavement parking ban started back in '74.
In most other places it remains a grey area for sure.
This leads to selfish exploitation in too many a case.
So *all* UK offenders should have a punishment to face.

Happy Birthday Bobby

Happy Birthday Bobby or 'SuperBob' to some!
A special day in Heaven, lots of birthday fun.
When I close my eyes, sometimes *I* am there!
In my dreamy moments, time with you I share.
All our love and wishes up to Heaven we send.
From your loving family and every single friend.
Heaven I know is distant, hidden from our view.
A magical, secret palace, is where I picture you!
Distance is no object, we love you just the same.
As today I picture 10 candles in my Angels name.

New Day

I looked up to the sky, I saw a beautiful day.
Nothing I could see would take the Sun away.
But a dark cloud appeared, devilish in shape.
A sunny day was eclipsed, finding no escape.

Where do I go from here, all alone in the rain?
How long must a person suffer all this pain?
Loved ones surround me, always there for me.
But an end to this battle one day I long to see.

How long I wonder for my new day to come?
When once again I will see and feel the Sun.
Today the sky is beautiful, radiant and bright.
Is this my new day, prayer answered overnight?

Ebbed Away

Driving for me is becoming a chore.
I can't really say I enjoy it anymore.
Necessity means a car I have to own.
When not in work, I leave it at home.

I love to walk, exercise and fresh air.
Avoiding drivers with their angry stare.
Driving standards, I've noticed decline.
Too often I see unpunished road crime.

Snarling brakes and red lights to beat.
Danger lurks in every road and street.
More speeding drivers I see by the day.
My driving pleasure all but ebbed away.

The Non Badge Holder 'Blue Badge Limp'

People think they have it off to a tee!
But a laughing stock they are to see.
A few variations, all with the one aim.
With added 'winces' part of fake pain.

It's not hard to master, their little trick.
To look unbalanced, in need of a stick.
To appear a little shaky, mobility poor.
They 'struggle' from car to shop door.

A couple of 'limps' for an added effect.
Fooling nobody with their non-defect!
But once in the shop a miraculous cure.
Suddenly they're not disabled no more!

But the Lazarus moment, alas is short.
Their ailment returns it's safe to report.
As on returning to their car right on cue.
A 'blue badge limp' once again they do!

Stop The World

The 2 fingers on a clock only move one way.
And second by second they eat into the day.
You can be sure following each day is night.
That's how God wants it, so it must be right.

There's a day on the calendar, you can't ring.
Yet on that Autumn day God's birds still sing.
Has God forgotten about you, I don't think so?
You want the World to stop, but God says no.

You have so much love to receive and to give.
That's why your one life you must try and live.
Time can't be turned back, it can't stand still.
Because God's time is a healer, and heal it will.

INDICATE !!

I notice it more every night and day.
No indicators used even where kids play.
Direction of vehicles we are left to guess.
Inconsiderate drivers, couldn't care less.
Cars can injure or kill even at low speed.
Always indicate when an obvious need.
Turning corners without it making it clear.
Endangers life when pedestrians are near.

Today The Bird is Blue

The famous Liver Bird, in the Liverpool sky.
A guardian of our City, protecting from a high.
It appears on the jersey of the team in red.
Thousands will appear wherever kopites tread.
Found all over the City, a landmark everyone.
They proudly remind me of what City I am from.
But they often lack colour, I look at some today.
I see Liver Birds of green, gold, black and grey.
But today is Bobby's day, so this is what to do.
Every Liver Bird you see today, picture it in blue!

Those Lenient Years

Justice campaigns started a few years ago.
But the Parliamentary process can be so slow.
Now great news announced for all our sake.
Campaigners' hard work, a difference to make.

Past sentences have been soft, that's a fact.
Now with tougher powers, the courts must act.
Dangerous drivers have often got off scott free.
Our 'hands were tied' excuses we would see.

So many bereaved families let down by the law.
So wrong and hopefully won't happen anymore.
Now a lifetime in jail these drivers could face.
I believe that should've always been the case.

A one sided legal system in serious road crime.
Offenders escaping punishment time after time.
Those lenient days that caused such a storm.
I hope have gone forever, no longer the norm.

Killer drivers spend an average of 4 years in jail.
Anguished families sickened with this system fail.
The law needed updating, an overhaul overdue.
But in future, Judges must now play their part too.

Winter Weather

A wheelchair can't compete with 2 strong feet.
So watch where you park in snow, ice or sleet.
Don't go stealing what doesn't belong to you.
In poor winter weather this is particularly true

Don't be a lazy driver, no excuse, no 'ifs or but'
You can manage in slippy conditions underfoot.
Consider those for whom that's not the case.
So don't encroach or steal a blue badge space.

If you do, it shows what sort of person you are.
So in winter time think where you park your car.
Disrespectful drivers still do it most of the time.
They should all face charges of a parking crime.

Support RoadPeace

Please support RoadPeace any way you can.
Like those who have walked, rode or swam.
Or just do whatever you like, it's your choice.
Share your awareness, don't be a lone voice.

Be creative and imaginative, have some fun!
And everything helps to raise essential income.
Organise social events, raffle prizes and such.
Everything you do will be appreciated so much!

Writing this little poetry book is what I chose.
And with these final words, this book I close.
A book written with every road victim in mind.
Though difficult at times the right words to find.

Nothing To Gain

Don't let this be a losing battle, words to be in vain.
Every day I see more accidents, everyday more pain.
Increasing number of drivers on mobile devices I see.
Don't let this be a losing battle, just don't let that be.
Every speed limit broken, injury or a life it might take.
Then follows a bereavement and a family heartbreak.
Ever seen such a heartache, I have, hence this rhyme.
Destroyed lives, a living nightmare suffered every time.
Speed kills, speed can ruin lives, speeding can maim.
Drive safely every journey, in speeding nothing to gain.

Angel Boy

Hello Mum a quick word from me.
Heaven is sound, all Sun and sea!
But if I want, I can also find snow!
I discover magic everywhere I go!

I send you signs; are they plain?
That little Robin flew in my name!
So don't worry about me as I'm ok.
We'll share cuddles again one day.

Dreams for now, we'll make them do.
As every dream up here comes true!
So please smile Mum, life's to enjoy.
With all my love, your little Angel boy.

SUPERBOB Books and Free School Assemblies by Jude Lennon
Book 1 https://thebobbycollerantrust.org.uk/product/superbob/
Book 2 https://thebobbycollerantrust.org.uk/product/s-t-o-p/

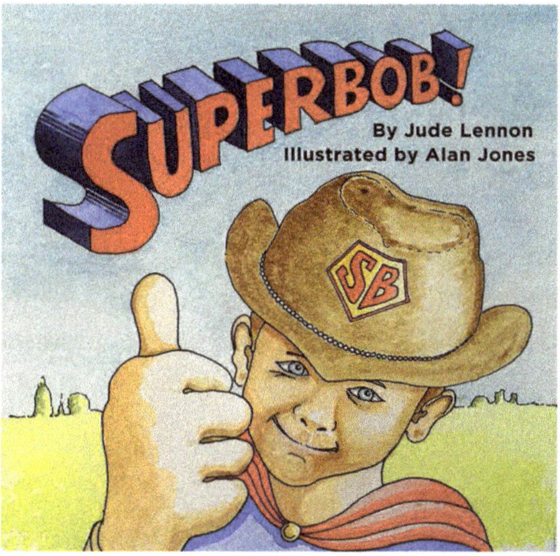

Free SUPERBOB road safety Primary school assemblies, to book an assembly for your school please email Jude at littlelambphonics@gmail.com

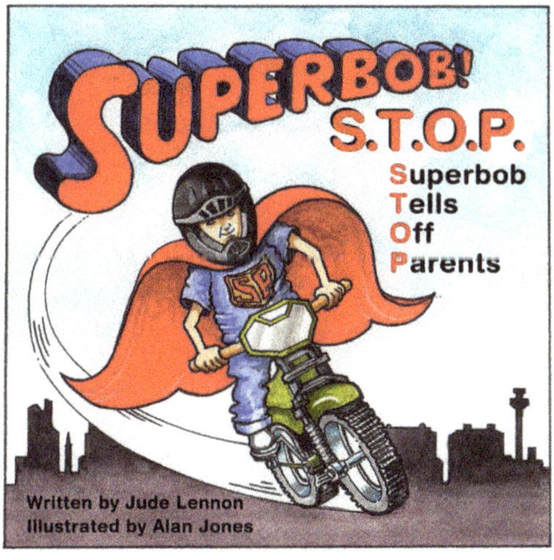

Acknowledgments

All digital images enhanced, resized and edited for this publication by Oliver and Jenny at http://www.facebook.com/PhotoFirstAidUK, thank you also for all the advice they kindly offered me along the way.
Front/Back Cover Design Oliver and Jenny
Front cover picture kindly provided by Janette Jones (with thanks also to Robin Jones)
RoadPeace Sculptor E-mail: tom.murphy@talk21.com
Many thanks to my brother Jon and sister Bernadette for their help and support and also to my daughters Emma and Rachel for their advice and input.

Other publications by the author
Hillsborough 20 Years On...ISBN 9781906823153
Justice Call...ISBN 9781906823283
The Nightmare of Hillsborough...ISBN 9781906828498
25 Years of Hillsborough Pain...ISBN 9781906823979
Hillsborough Our Greatest Victory...ISBN 9781786238825
Road Safety and Awareness (In Memory of Bobby Colleran) ...ISBN 9781786238825

All proceeds from the above publications are donated to various charities and good causes.

Please try and support these 2 wonderful charities...
RoadPeace...www. www.roadpeace.org
The Bobby Colleran Trust...https://thebobbycollerantrust.org.uk

All poems by Mike Bartram...dandy.77@hotmail.co.uk
To Joanne and David Colleran and Pauline Fielding I would like to say their strength and dedication is my inspiration, God bless and look after you.